Brain Code.

The Benchmark of Decoding the Brain.

One Against which all are Evaluated.

By David Gomadza

The First Global President.

ISBN: 978-1-4477-6925-5

This is volume V in the Thoughts to Word or Audio series.

This must be read after Volume I to IV.

FREE DOWNLOADS FROM GOOLE PLAY BOOKS

https://play.google.com/store/books/details/David_G omadza_Thoughts_To_Word_Or_Audio?id=q2xmE AAAQBAJ&gl=GB

https://play.google.com/store/books/details/David_G omadza_Decoding_Thoughts_and_Inner_Voice_Ex?i d=qi1qEAAAQBAJ&gl=GB

https://play.google.com/store/books/details/David_G omadza_DATESTAMP_28_March_2022_Thoughts_ to?id=rrizEAAAQBAJ&gl=GB

https://play.google.com/store/books/details/David_G omadza_Genesis_Brain_Language_Construction?id= WKm1EAAAQBAJ&gl=GB

Brain Code. The Benchmark of Decoding the Brain.

Brain Code. The Benchmark of Decoding the Brain.

DEDICATION

To one of the most advanced stages of human development.

ACKNOWLEDGMENTS

That time has come when we speak through thoughts.

Brain Code. The Benchmark of Decoding the Brain.

BRAIN CODE.

The Benchmark of Decoding the Brain. One Against which all are Evaluated.

The reason why it took so long to have a breakthrough in decoding thoughts is the sheer fact that there was no gold standard of decoding the brain against which one measures the progress and success of his or her project. This book is now the reference point to see how far you are in decoding the brain.

This book should be the gold standard for decoding thoughts. I am not saying that this is the perfect solution to the decoding of the brain problem. No. But this shall be the litmus test. Surely, we need to improve further to methods where you just place an EEG device on top of someone's head and know straight away what that person is thinking. But being realistic about the issue means we must start somewhere. This is where to start. I believe my method will help to achieve that stage. My method will act as a guiding benchmark where everyone serious about decoding the brain will have to check if they are in the right direction.

My plan.

The need for a comprehensive approach.

This method is tried, tested, and evaluated. The method works. But I know it works because we have predefined parameters through the language we constructed. But I believe this is the first stage. Even when it comes to speaking, language construction was critical. I have done my best to construct a language that we can use as a guideline, especially for this crude early stage of brain decoding. But the aim is to combine this method with what the current research is trying to do by just working from the outside of the body. In the end, the aim is to have the brain language I have constructed supplemented by actual acoustic wave sounds that match that word, verb, or noun.

We also need an MEG, EEG, and fMRI, that matches the language constructed and the acoustic wave.

On top of that, we need an electromagnetic or light wave of the same word when we speak normally.

In the end, we must compare all these to find what we can learn from all this.

Is it true that the brain is too complicated for humans to understand? Can we wait for machines to decode the brain for us?

So, what makes the brain so difficult for humans to decipher?

What are the most common problems encountered in decoding the brain?

1. Difficulties in recording and decoding the brain.

2. Difficulties in understanding and knowing how speech is handled by the brain that is how it is stored and processed.

3. Difficulties in recording thoughts and their translation to a language we can understand.

First, we do not need machines to understand the brain. I can and have decoded the brain. I will address all the challenges one by one.

Brain language construction.

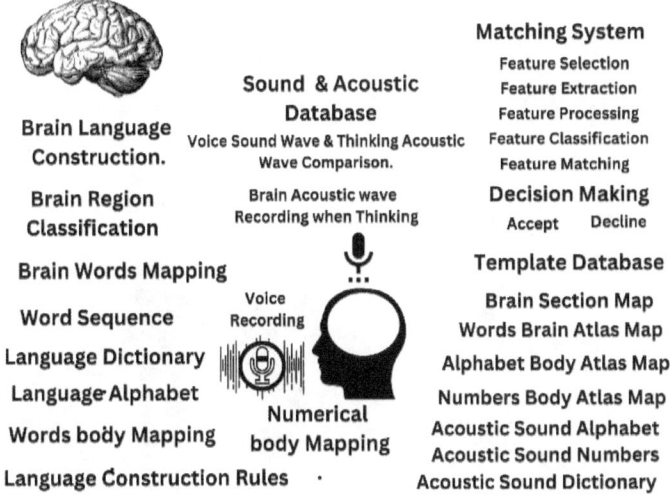

Brain Language Construction.

Brain Region Classification

Brain Words Mapping

Word Sequence

Language Dictionary

Language Alphabet

Words body Mapping

Language Construction Rules

Sound & Acoustic Database

Voice Sound Wave & Thinking Acoustic Wave Comparison.

Brain Acoustic wave Recording when Thinking

Voice Recording

Numerical body Mapping

Matching System

Feature Selection

Feature Extraction

Feature Processing

Feature Classification

Feature Matching

Decision Making

Accept   Decline

Template Database

Brain Section Map

Words Brain Atlas Map

Alphabet Body Atlas Map

Numbers Body Atlas Map

Acoustic Sound Alphabet

Acoustic Sound Numbers

Acoustic Sound Dictionary

I have argued in volume IV that to understand something we must know the basic surrounding of that something. If it is a normal language, we only understand what is said after learning it, its English language construction pattern, and rules, etc. Likewise, we must first construct a brain language we will use against all tests we will do. Refer to volume IV for the details. But I will expand on brain language construction.

In this book volume V, I will advocate and argue that we need a system of construction language and rules of the brain language that will make it possible to know exactly what a person is thinking at a specific time and place.

This is the first time you will ever hear this. Any word must have **seven** different expressions, forms, or definitions. This is the only way we will be able to understand the brain thoughts. You can call this David's Seven Expressions Golden Rule of decoding the brain.

The seven expressions or forms of any given word.

Any given word MUST have 7 expressions /forms/ definitions

English or any Language	Voice Sound wave Language	EEG fMRI Scan Language	Light/ Acoustic Wave Language	Brain Language Sequence	Body Alphabet Map Language	Binary /Body Number Map Language

Clap

Thoughts to recording device
Thoughts to word or audio
Word to numbers
Numbers to binary converter or calculator
Binary to device commands convertor
Success Brain Computer Interface

Front   Back
Mirror Image But in reverse

1. The written form in English or any another language.
2. The voice sound pattern waveform.
3. Spectrogram representation includes scans from EEG, fMRI, PET, MEG etc.
4. Light or acoustic waveform.
5. Brain language sequence.
6. Human body alphabet map.
7. Human body binary and number map language.

This is the only way we can be able to interpret what someone is thinking at any given time and space. Anyone who says otherwise does not fully understand the amazing thing the human body is.

The written form in English or other language.

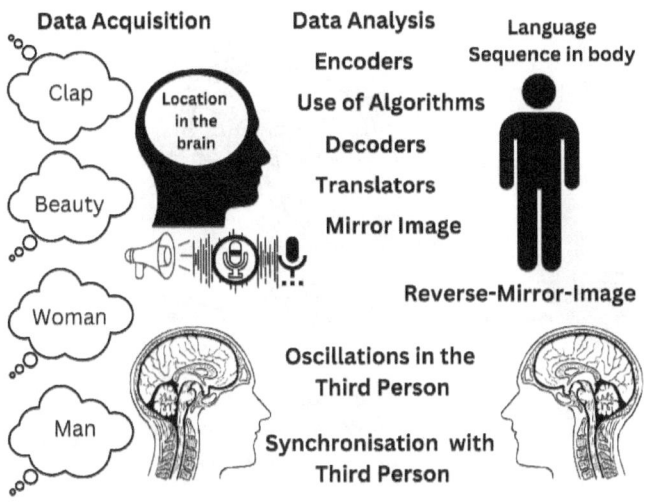

We only understand spoken English because we constructed the language and know the rules surrounding that language so that when a person speaks. We can easily understand what they are saying. Imagine a young baby listening to someone speaking in a language he has not learned yet, surely you cannot expect that child to know what the speaker is saying.

To the brain language, all these today's scientists are like that child who does not know what English language is. Of course, the child can repeat the words she or he is hearing but he or she does not understand what that means straight away until he or she first understands the language. Understanding the *language* first then becomes the key to decoding the brain.

The English language has an alphabetic order from a to z and all these letters are twenty-six in total. There are rules for constructing sentences etc. The brain arranges all words in the brain to specific areas in the brain. I have divided the brain into four major regions.

Aerial View of the head

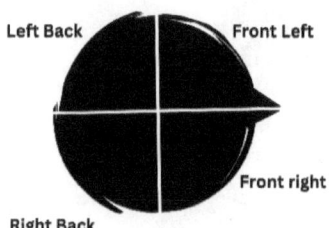

The head is divided into four regions.

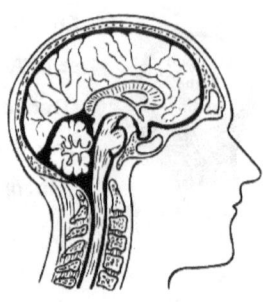

Areas of the brain are noted for what they are responsible for

1. The front right.
2. The left front.
3. The right back
4. The left back.

The brain has a clever storing system of words for easy access. The brain first stores words in specific parts of the brain for easy access and retrieval. This is critical in understanding thoughts.

How the brain stores the alphabetical order.

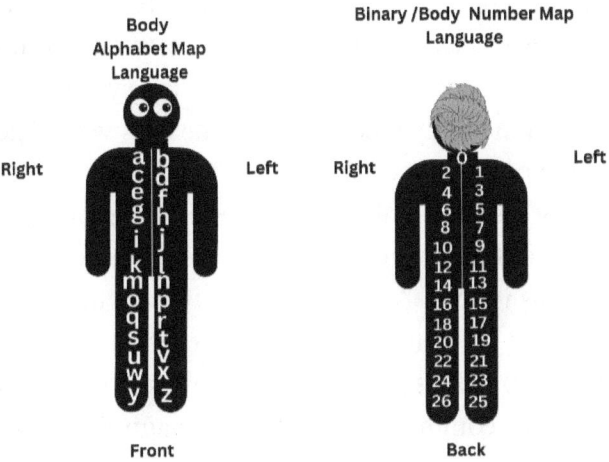

The brain points to the region and side of the brain where it stores the words first as a reference or check digit. This is part of the language sequence that enables the brain to store so many words and process things faster. Any letter of the alphabetic order has two sequence points.

1. The part the brain first points to when someone thinks about this letter or when the brain hears this letter.
2. The specific point of the letter of the alphabet where it is stored on the body.

So, let us look at all the 26 letters of the alphabet one by one.

A.

This is the first letter of the English alphabetical order. The brain when it first hears this word will save this letter using a sequence as a check digit and the actual place to find the word. This is a reference point to make sure that the letter is stored correctly.

7

To the brain, the letter A is a reference in the front right of the brain. This place acts as the check digit for reference purposes and ease of access. The second aspect of the sorting system is to find a specific point on the body where to store these as well. The second storing system point is not on the brain. This is stored on the right side of the body just below the collarbone. I will explain later why the body must do this. In short, this is the fastest way that makes the brain think as it does. Above all, this will help the brain know what the person is going to think, say next or think about. Secondly, this will help it predict what the person is about to say so that it sends motor commands in advance. Imagine thinking about touching something and doing it in seconds. This helps the brain act faster at lightning speeds.

So, in short, A as the first word of the alphabetical order which is a letter that has two reference points in the human body.

1. The right front side of the brain.
2. The right side of the body on the collarbone.

Ladies and gentlemen this is your first brain language construction lesson.

So, on the body; A is stored in the front of the brain and right collarbone.

Now you can create a computer algorithm or interface and enter this information as the definition of A to the brain.

So now if you touch the collarbone first and the right front side of the brain [theoretically] the brain will know you are talking about A. So, it will point to the right side and the collarbone.

Tell me what you have noticed about what I said above?

Anyone?

The brain listens to the reverse mirror image. Imagine looking at yourself in the mirror. What you write or say is read by your 'mirror' in reverse. Above I pointed to the collarbone first and the right side of the brain. This will make the brain know what you are talking about as the brain takes your last input as its first input.

Your last input was pointing to the right front part of the brain. So, the brain will point first to this front part and then the collarbone.

Another rule is that the brain language has double the meaning. This is in relation to the fact I mentioned above that every word on earth must have at least seven expressions or forms. Any letter or word to the brain can be expressed in terms of words and letters and numbers.

Let us look at how the brain stores the alphabetic order and the numbers in the body.

Over centuries the body has found an easy way to store the alphabetic letters and numbers in the body. For this book, we will only look at numbers 1 to 26 that correspond to the alphabetical order.

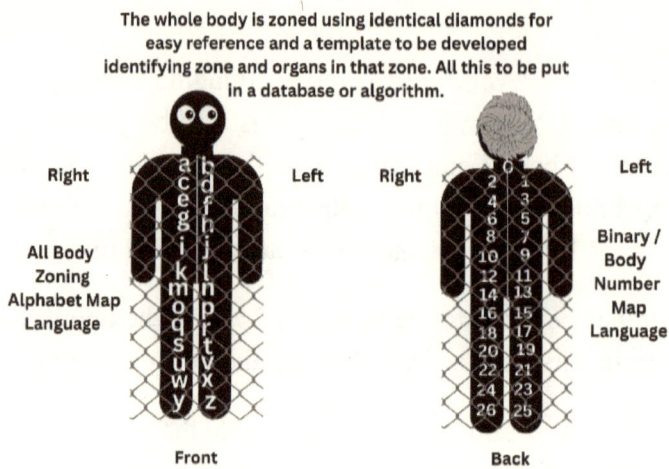

The whole body is zoned using identical diamonds for easy reference and a template to be developed identifying zone and organs in that zone. All this to be put in a database or algorithm.

The body stores to the right side of the body or the left going down this applies both to the alphabetical letters and numbers. I explained the reasons why it does this. So, we know where A as a letter is stored by the body. On the collarbone.

If A is on the right side so the next letter B must be opposite so on the left side. That means C will be on the right below A and D on the left side below B. So, A to Z are stored on the body down to the feet.

Numbers 1 to 26 are stored on the back of the body. 1 is stored on the right back of the body. 2 on the left back of the body and so on until 26 on the back of the left foot.

0 is the back neck of the body.

This is critical as we will find out later that this will make it possible to convert words into numbers and therefore into binary. the computer or machine language something all researchers have missed out on. Thanks to me, I will give you everything on a plate simply because I am the man to understand all this.

Now we look at words and how the brain deals with these.

To the brain, most words fall into any of the 4 regions.

1. Right front.
2. Right back.
3. Left front.
4. Right back.

The brain distributes words according to gender as well. Man, for example, is stored in the right side of the brain whereas woman is stored, the left back side of the brain. Volume III and IV have a lot of examples of how the brain stores these words.

Most of the words the brain uses daily are stored in the right backside of the brain. We look at 100 commonly used English verbs.

Aerial View of the head

An EEG 10-10 International system can be superimposed on top and all linked to the zones created below

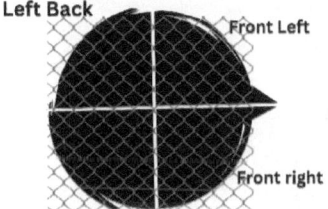

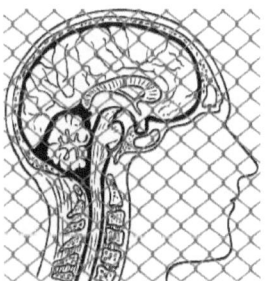

The whole head is number-marked, zoned and color coded using 4 colors; gold, blue, purple and scarlet and equal diamond shapes

Words that are stored in the right back of the brain.

1. be
2. have
3. Do is stored in the left back side of the brain.
4. say
5. go
6. can
7. get
8. would
9. make
10. know
11. will
12. think
13. take
14. see
15. come
16. could
17. want
18. Look is stored in the left side of the brain.
19. use
20. find
21. give
22. tell
23. work
24. may
25. should
26. call
27. try
28. ask
29. need
30. Feel
31. become
32. leave
33. put
34. mean
35. keep

36. let
37. begin
38. seem
39. help
40. Tall is stored in the left back.
41. turn
42. start
43. might
44. show
45. hear
46. play
47. run
48. move
49. like
50. Live

51. believe
52. hold
53. bring
54. happen
55. must
56. write
57. provide
58. sit
59. stand
60. lose
61. pay
62. meet
63. include
64. continue
65. set
66. lcarn
67. change
68. lead
69. understand
70. watch
71. follow

72. stop
73. create
74. speak
75. read
76. allow
77. add
78. spend
79. grow
80. open
81. walk
82. win
83. offer
84. remember
85. love
86. consider
87. appear
88. buy
89. wait
90. serve
91. die
92. send
93. expect
94. build
95. stay
96. fall
97. cut
98. reach
99. Kill.

100. remain

100 commonly used nouns.

1. time
2. year
3. people
4. way

5.   day
6.   man
7.   thing
8.   Women is stored in the left backside of the brain.
9.   life
10. child
11. World is stored in the left back side of the brain.
12. school
13. state
14. family
15. student
16. group
17. country
18. problem
19. hand
20. part
21. place
22. case
23. week
24. company
25. system
26. program
27. question
28. work
29. government
30. number
31. night
32. point
33. home
34. Water

35. room
36. Mother is tired in the left backside of the brain.
37. area
38. money
39. story
40. fact

41. month
42. Lot is stored in the left side of the brain.
43. right
44. study
45. book
46. eye
47. job
48. word
49. business
50. issue
51. side
52. kind
53. head
54. house
55. service
56. friend
57. father
58. power
59. hour
60. game
61. line
62. end
63. member
64. law
65. car
66. city
67. community
68. name
69. the president is stored at the center of the brain.
70. team
71. minute
72. idea
73. Kid is tired in the left side of the brain.
74. body
75. information
76. back
77. Parents are stored at the center of the brain.

78. face
79. others
80. level
81. office
82. door
83. health
84. person
85. art
86. war
87. history
88. party
89. result
90. change
91. morning
92. reason
93. research
94. Girl is stored in the left back of the brain.
95. guy
96. moment
97. air
98. teacher
99. force
100. education

1. Personal Pronouns / Subject Pronouns

- I
- we
- you (singular and plural)
- he
- She is stored in the left back side of the brain.
- it
- the

2. Object Pronouns

- me

- us
- you (singular and plural)
- She is stored in the left back side of the brain.
- him
- it
- them

3. Possessive Pronouns

- mine
- ours
- yours (singular and plural)
- hers is stored in the left back side of the brain.
- his
- theirs

- my
- our
- your
- She is stored in the left back side of the brain.
- his
- their

4. Reflexive Pronouns

- myself
- yourself
- herself is stored in the left back side of the brain.
- himself
- itself
- ourselves
- yourselves
- themselves

5. Intensive Pronouns

myself

- yourself
- herself is stored in the left back side of the brain.
- himself
- itself
- ourselves
- yourselves
- themselves

6. Indefinite Pronouns

- all
- another
- any
- anybody
- anyone
- anything
- both
- each
- either
- everybody
- everyone
- everything
- few
- many
- most
- neither
- nobody
- none
- no one
- nothing
- one
- other
- others
- several
- some
- somebody
- someone

- something
- such

7. Demonstrative Pronouns

- such
- that
- these
- this
- those

8. Interrogative Pronouns

- what
- whatever
- which
- whichever
- who
- whoever
- whom
- whomever
- whose

9. Relative Pronouns

- as
- that
- what
- whatever
- which
- whichever
- who
- whoever
- whom
- whomever
- whose

10. Archaic Pronouns

- it is stored in the left back side of the dead.
- Thy is stored in the left back side
- Thine is stored in the left back side.
- Ye is stored on the left back side.

As a rule, most of the words used every day are stored in the right backside of the brain. Words to do with God and women are stored in the left back side of the brain. As a rule, the brain points to the side of the brain in which a word is stored first. If you say, man. The brain will show lots of activity on MRI scans on the right backside of the brain. If you say woman, then on the left side as the first sequence. There are other words like president that are stored at the center of the brain.

Dealing with numbers.

When it comes to numbers the brain stores things a bit differently.

When it comes to numbers the brain first points to one as a written word. Then to the actual place in the body where it stores the number.

1.

Right back side of the brain and the right back shoulder of the body.

2.

Left-back side of the brain and the left back shoulder of the body.

3.

Right-back side of the brain and right back shoulder of the body.

4.

Left-back side of the brain and left back shoulder of the body.

5.

Right-back side of the brain and right back shoulder of the body.

26.

Right-back side of the brain and right back foot of the right leg.

For some words, the body points to all the meanings of the word. Means all expressions, all forms of that word. Let us take clapping as a word.

Clap is a four-letter word.

The body will point to the place of the body where it stores this word. The right back side of the brain. Secondly, a word is made up of four letters. c, l, a, and p.

So automatically the language construction will mean that the brain must spell clap to you as well. If you say clap the software must be designed in such a manner that after pointing to the place in the right back of the brain. It must trace the sequence of the words that make up clap. Using the alphabetical order body map, we can see that c is 2 places down from the top and on the right side of the body just below A.

So, this is the first sequence of the word clap.

Secondly, L is on the left side of the body and the 6th place down from the first letter B on that side.

Thirdly, the sequence points to A. This is the first letter on the right side of the body.

Fourthly we need P. This is the 8th letter down from B.

So, saying clap as a word will automatically trigger the brain to point to the right backside of the brain and as the first point of the sequence.

Then to C as a point on the body.

Followed by pointing to L, then A, and lastly to P's position on the body map.

But Clap is also a verb that involves movement, sounds, and vibrations as an action or command. If I say clap as a person you do not point to places in the body like what the brain does but you clap.

So again, as part of the 7 expressions and forms of any word you can write or define clap just by clapping.

Putting your hands together and clapping to produce the clap sound that is absorbed by the ground as sound waves.

When creating the language of the brain this must also be incorporated as part of the 7 forms of any given word.

Now if we are programming the brain language of the word clap. This must also be included. So, all the sequences will include.

1. The back side of the brain word to where the English written form is stored.

2. The spelling as positions in the body; c, l, a, and p.
3. The clapping as a command. That is the command given to motor neurons sent to hands through the elbows. So, the language to be programmed must point to the right-hand elbow and then the left-hand elbow that sends commands to hands to join and clap to produce the clap noises. So, the motion of joining hands together forms the sequence. When hand joins and claps; a sound is released that is lost generally to the ground. So, the downward motion is part of the definition of clap. After clapping the hands are lowered down, which is a form of deflation.

So, in short, these are the commands and actions the brain language is expected to show when someone thinks about clapping.

1. Right back side of the brain.
2. Second place down to the right of the body below A.
3. 6 places down on the left side to L
4. First position on the right to A.
5. Then to the 8th place on the left to P.
6. Then to right elbow [as a brain command given to motor neurons sent to elbows].
7. Then to the left elbow.
8. Hands are brought together, and they clap, and a sound is released.
9. The released sound escapes into the ground illustrated by a downward motion.
10. After clapping hands are lowered and the body deflates.

But I said every word as a rule, call it David's 7 meanings rule; every word must have 7 meanings. So far, we have 3 out of the seven.

1. The written form of clap.
2. The alphabetical order forms on the body as letters of the alphabet.
3. We have the brain sequence language of the physical way to clap.
4. We can use the letters to get the corresponding number form of the word clap.

The Numerical and binary form of clap as a word.

What we did with the alphabetical order of placing it either left or right side of the body can be done to numbers but since this is a different system [words to numbers] we can put this to the back and use the laws of inverse proportions to link the word to the numerical representations.

Mirror image as part of the brain language construction.

I explained in volume IV that everything in the universe rotates around itself or something else. I also stated that you must consider the four regions of the brain as separate entities with rotational properties. So, the right back side of the brain must be viewed theoretically as able to rotate separately independent of the left front or the right front or the left back. This is part of the rule of brain language construction. That means when for example the right side is 'rotating' that means it takes the form of a circle. Assuming we slice the middle of a circle into two sides and place a mirror in between, whatever is on one side is reflected in the other half but in a different form. In other words, whatever is in the left half of the brain side we are talking about; is also on the other side but in a different format or is read from back to front.

In this case if one is looking in the mirror. The word clap on the body will be on the opposite side of the body because the mirror image is facing us. So, the correct side on the body that represents clap will be as follows.

The front right side of the body as words is equivalent to the left back side of the body as numbers.

That means the left front side of the body is equivalent to the right backside of the body.

Therefore, clap as a number is.

C = 3.

L = 12 [6 positions down x 2]

A = 1.

P = 16 [8 positions down x 2].

As a digit clap =3.12.1.16

Binary numbers.

We will need binary number conversions.

CLAP as a number is 312116.

In binary using a binary converter is [hex to Binary] 3212116 = 11000100100001000010110.

Now we have four out of the seven words to express a word.

Sound Wave as spoken word.

This is the easy one. Simply download a free voice recorder from

Google Play Apps and install it on your phone. Now simply record yourself saying the word clap. Get the mp3 player.

Download and install NCH Mixpad Multitrack.

https://www.nch.com.au/mixpad/index.html?theme=multitrack&kw=multitrack%20recorder&gclid=Cj0KCQjwiZqhBhCJARIsACHHEH9PIcNOHeHViPK7FWc1nH-JTNPuAfq3korLuTIczYKgezQo5gxpLZcaAojwEALw_wcB

See instructions in volume IV and amplify the track then export it then change its name.

Now you will need NCH Wavepad software.

https://www.nch.com.au/wavepad/index.html?ns=true&kw=wavepad&gclid=Cj0KCQjwiZqhBhCJARIsACHHEH9cT-tZYuxVf4Ic8BDPQ9tA54WgjCmdGqN8ILZolMhhZuCyqJXWZIgaAr9kEALw_wcB

Download and install.

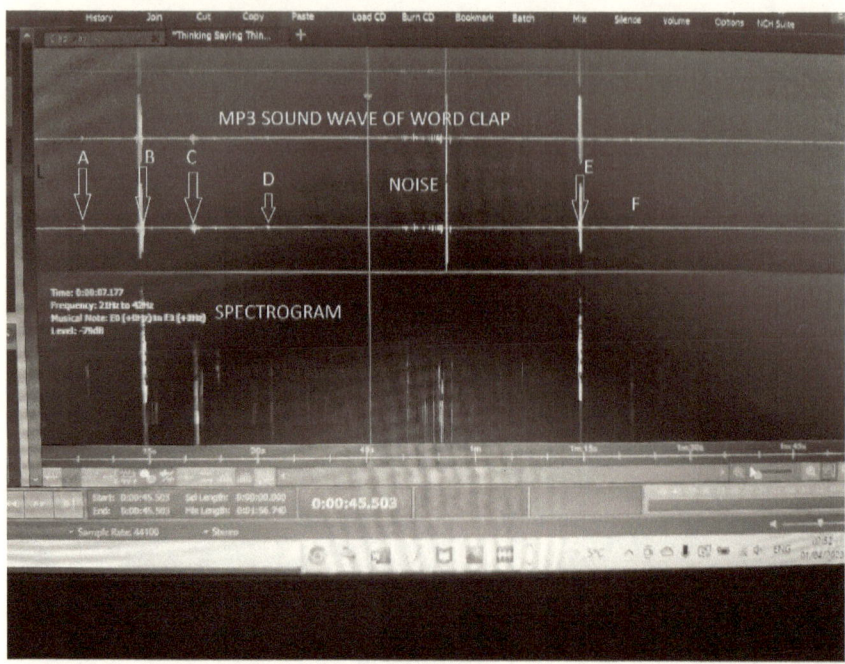

The above wave is when a person thinks the word clap. Then after a few seconds then actually says the word then remains quiet then repeats the word clap; speaking this word then keeps quiet.

We have included a spectrogram of the sound wave. That means so far, we have almost 5 versions of the word clap.

1. The written English or any language.

2. The body alphabetical order map.

3. The binary and number map on the body.

4. The sound voice [spoken word]

5. Now the spectrogram version of the word.

But as you will discover after explaining we already have the light or acoustic wave above, but it is hidden. I must point out which one is the acoustic or light wave.

That means 6 versions already. Is not it wonderful doing doubles without knowing it?

A: in the picture above is the brain language of how it recognizes the word clap. The person simply thinks about the word without speaking and a voice recorder through a powerful speaking and spinning rotary propeller pick its signal up on the recording. But like I explained in volume IV if not amplified it will not show on the wave or spectrogram. Most play at -45db.

The body uses mirror image systems. Whatever is in one part of the brain it is also on the other mirror part of the brain but in a different form. Hence my method insists that one must define all seven forms of the word first before even thinking about knowing what one is thinking. So, the basis of our brain language is the fact that any given word must be expressed in seven different forms

Thinking produces electromagnetic waves that are converted or amplified by the magnets in the rotary propeller and speakers to acoustic. The body replaces the person's thoughts about the word clap by producing an acoustic version. This is the spike on the wave. If you program the brain language correctly and link it to decoders and BCIs on the screen automatically the word clap will start flashing.

Brain Code. The Benchmark of Decoding the Brain.

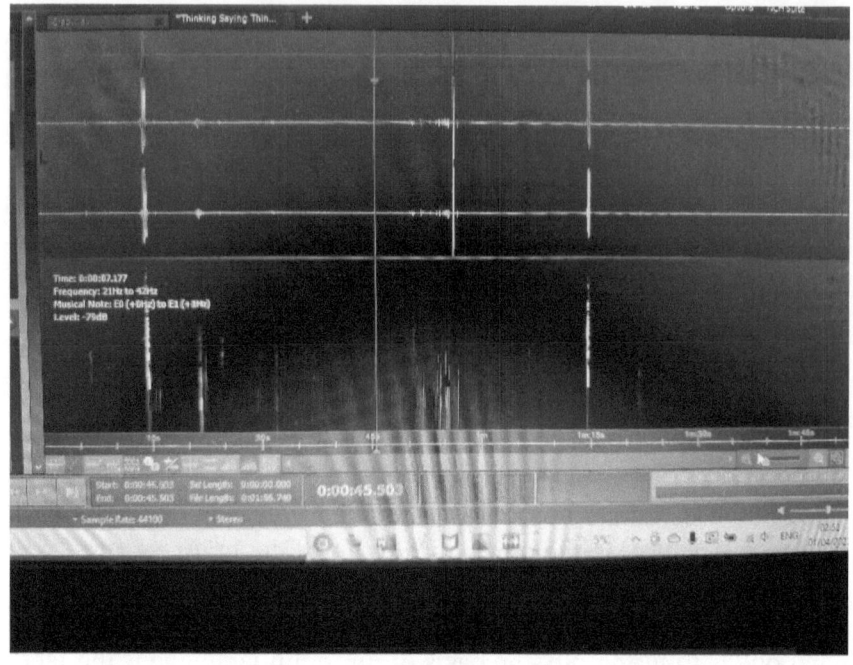

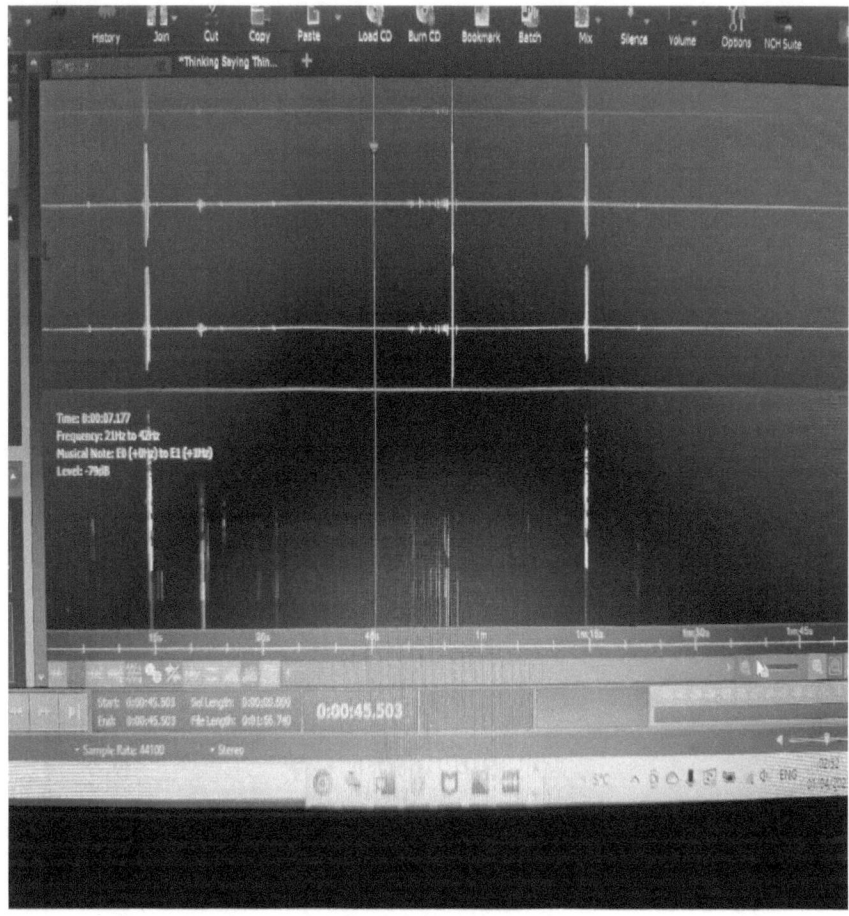

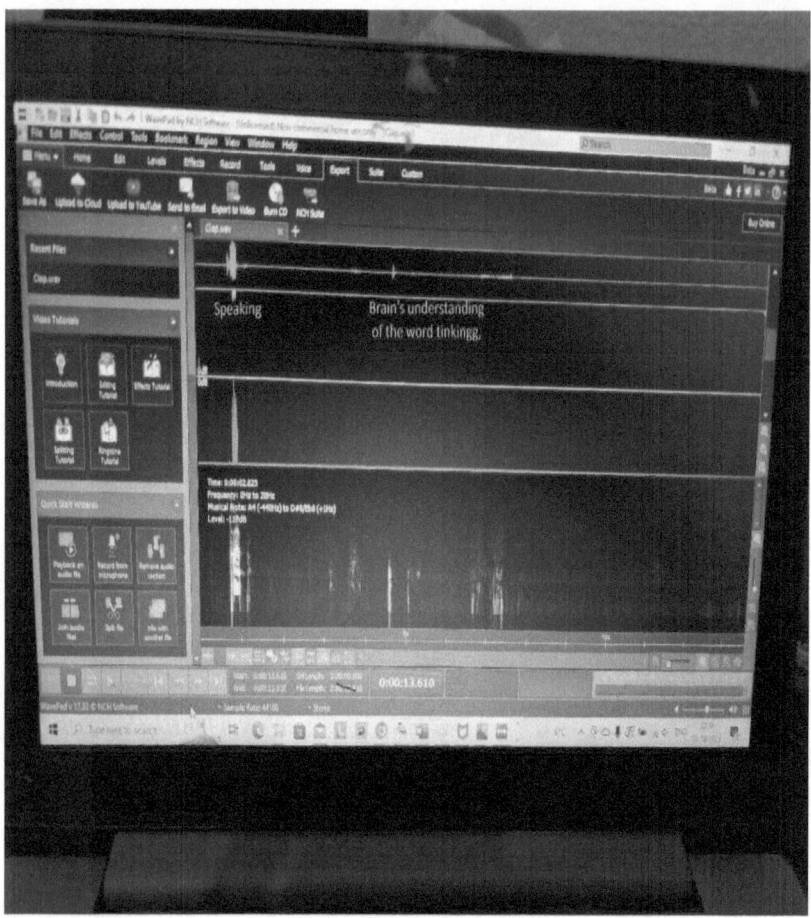

The image below is the second speaking of the word clap with a lower voice than at the beginning.

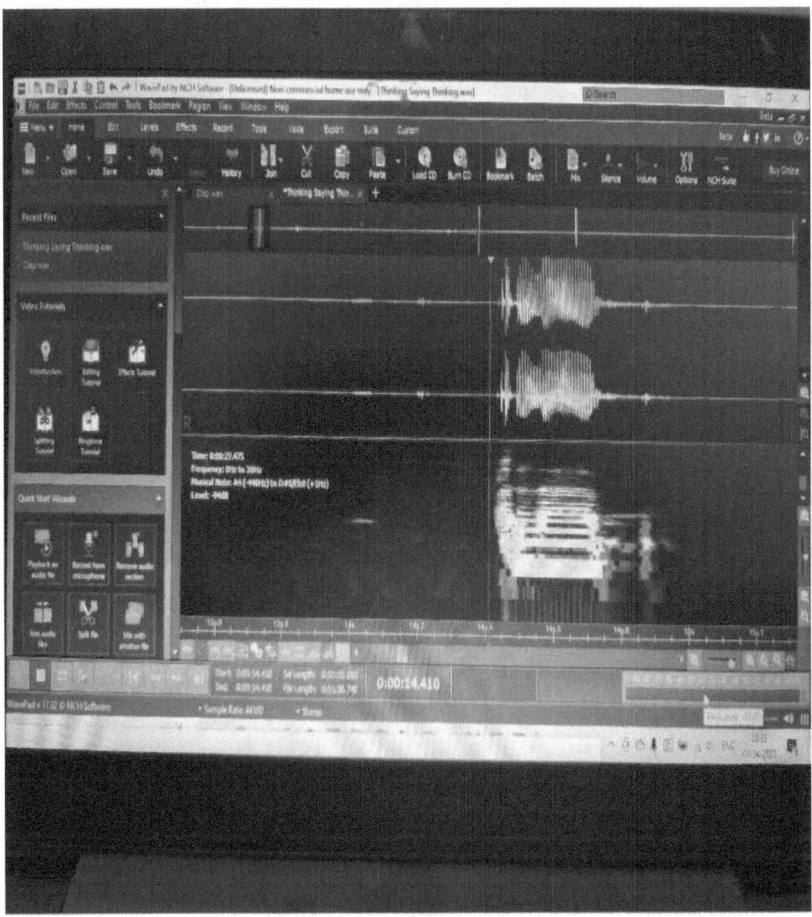

After expanding waves both the sound wave and the spectrogram you can see clearly the two other expressions or forms of the word clap.

This will be the same for every person if they are using the same language.

So, we have a spectrogram definition of the word clap. That orange or fire image above.

Below is the image of speaking out loud the word clap and the brain reproducing the same exact spectrogram.

B and E are the same. The word clap was spoken out in both instances.

So, to round up.

From beginning to A is the thinking part of the person without saying a word but thinking about the word clap.

The spike at A is the brain's processing of the word clap. The acoustic waveform is such that if it is replayed the brain will in reverse mode or other of the seven forms define the word clap.

This is the command needed to control any output devices etc.

B is the time the person spoke out loud the word clap.

I explained in the earlier volumes that the body has three systems all working together differently and all produce seven forms of any word which they all interpret the same but in different ways. Any word that is thought or spoken produces by-products which the other system uses to further produce a different version.

It is like the oxygen and carbon cycle. Humans need the oxygen which they use to produce carbon. Then the plants take the carbon to use and produce back oxygen.

After the person has spoken the word clap. The brain picks up this and converts it to acoustic which is replayed producing C and D.

In the picture above I included a noise section between D and E but in fact, this is not a noise it is another version of the word clap. This is the alphabetical mapping of the word on the body but for this volume, we will call it noise. I will expand in volume VI.

E is the repeat of the word clap speaking out louder but less than at point B. But the waves are the same. The spectrogram is identical, check the zoomed one below.

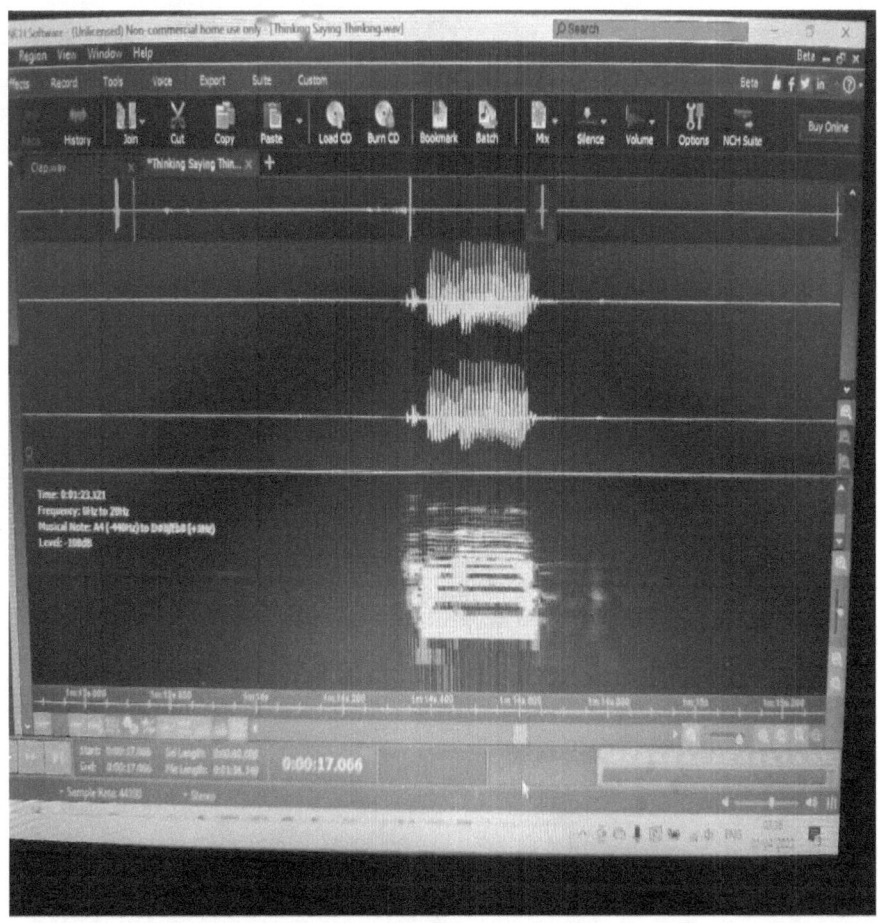

You can find this sound wave on SoundCloud click this link

https://soundcloud.com/david-gomadza

Then search for a track titled: Thinking Saying Thinking.wav

Watch the video on YouTube.

https://www.youtube.com/watch?v=6gLfsa0D8L4

Creating the acoustic alphabetical order.

Any alphabetical order has letters that make it. Letters that will become part and parcel of the language. So, if we make an acoustic language of the whole alphabetical order when someone is just thinking. That is a to z just thinking without any words and recording these. To use these to construct words from scratch is something that is possible.

So, I compiled all 26 letters of the thinking alphabet and uploaded them all on SoundCloud.

https://soundcloud.com/david-gomadza

Now as you know clap is a word made up of letters of the alphabet. It must also follow that we take our thinking alphabet and construct the word clap. It must be able to look and sound to the brain just like the word clap.

So, I took this to the test and the system recognizes the word clap just by constructing the word from the alphabetic order.

That means now at this stage we do not even need to know what the spectrogram or sound wave pattern looks like.

All we need now is the acoustic alphabetical order created just from someone's thoughts about this alphabet.

So now all you need is the alphabet on SoundCloud to construct any word the brain will understand and act upon.

Can decoding the brain be this easy? Why it took people so long?

Yes, it is easy, but the tricky part is to understand the language rules I formulated above. David's rule number one.

There are seven expressions, forms, and definitions for any given word.

So, the word of success is in obeying this critical rule and constructing seven versions of every single word.

Like always we must start with the position of the brain where the word is stored by the brain.

First is to start with easy four or three-letter words.

Using our thinking SoundCloud database

https://soundcloud.com/david-gomadza

So, we must also include this on SoundCloud as part of the language just thinking about the right backside of the brain where the word clap is stored.

But one thing I have noticed is the fact that when recording the alphabetical letters. The length of each letter is too long so if joined everything takes longer. A solution might be increasing the speed and the tempo or trimming the letters [acoustic or electromagnetic wave].

Or to re-record as short waves as possible so that when we join the letters the word will be easily understood. But it works.

We will also need to add the end of the word with a deflationary effect. If you raise your hands to clap after you finished clapping you lower both hands and your shoulders. In this brain language, this would signal the end of the action.

So, every word has a beginning and an end.

For most words, the beginning is the same. The right back side of the brain since most of the everyday words are stored there.

The end for some is the deflation effect or the shoulders down.

Now go to SoundCloud and search for C.L.A.P [one we constructed from the alphabet].

You will find out that the system or algorithm will be able to identify all the letters and their position in the body. So, we can use the alphabet to construct the acoustic version, the spectrogram, the body sequence, and the numeric or binary version of the word.

I will expand on this in volume VI.

There are other words the body does not store in the brain. Take legs for example the body will point straight to the legs as per our programming. So, we must program the software in such a way that if one thinks about the legs the body will point to the right leg first then the left leg and to some extent define what legs do. So, for walking that can be explained by tapping the bottom of the legs. Running can mean that tapping below the feet is faster. Etc.

For some actions that occur inside the brain like thinking the brain will still point to the right backside first as the place it stores the word. Then perform a three-dimensional [triangle] move in the brain to indicate where thinking happens. So first the tongue creates the bouncing off of words that trigger the thinking. This is interesting especially, considering that it is simply thinking without talking.

Above all, it proves also that when one is thinking or talking the

38

brain uses the same principles. Thinking is triggered by the same processes as talking. Words are still created in other versions. These bounce off the tongue to the area the brain stores these. To the right backside of the brain.

Ideally instantly the new version I believe the electromagnetic or now acoustic wave will bounce to the other half of the head meaning the left backside of the brain. That bounces off the word thinking but probably in a different version back to the tongue.

This explains why we hear voices in the head when one thinks silently.

How to construct the brain language that involves other creatures.

Animals must be represented differently. Most animals are four-legged beings. Birds are two-legged creatures. So, these two aspects can form part of the word definition, especially in sequencing.

So, a cat for example even though the word is stored in the same part of the brain. The right back side. To construct the programming language must point to the fact that it is a four-legged animal. To bend it down. One must press the right shoulder down. Then the left shoulder. Then the right back and the left back. That makes the animal bend down to a four-legged animal. So, a slight bending down effect can be part of the language. Now the animal has all its legs on the ground. So, this also can be part of the language. So right front leg. Left front leg. Right back leg and lastly the left back leg can all be part of the language.

But a cat has a tail. So, we can include the tail as part of the language. But most animals are like that so how do we distinguish a cat from a dog?

We can include the cat's whiskers as part of the sequence definition. On top of that, we can include the sound it makes to further distinguish it like that. A cat meows. So, this becomes part of the sequence definition of the cat.

The word bird is stored in the same part of the brain. Placing weight on the right shoulder and then the left shoulder will bend down the bird. But before that; one can also explain that a bird has wings by creating the opening of arms outward to represent this. A bending down means a bird, even if it flies, can walk on the ground with the right leg. Then the left leg. Standing straight after can also be part of the sequence to indicate flying as the bird flies off the ground.

The 7 expressions rule means every time someone says a word the system must express all seven forms in their different meanings and representations. Thinking about beauty will and must make the system and the body define beauty in seven different ways.

1. The written word is written down on a hand-held interface or a watch etc. I will explain in detail about synchronization. Ideally, all relevant instruments and devices must be synchronized even if we are not the person thinking about beauty. A printer or fax must also be connected to the system. So that when a person thinks about the word beauty. The print miles away will print the word beauty. A fax will fax that word. A phone will receive a text message with the name. A computer will have the word written on a screen.
2. The spectrogram of the word beauty will be printed or flashed on the software responsible for that etc.

3. The sound version is played deep in the ears of the listeners and the synchronized third parties. I will elaborate on this in volume VI.
4. The EEG, MEG, the fMRI, etc. will be printed and reflected on the machines responsible.
5. In the mirror image of the second person linked to the person the alphabet sequence of the word is played to this person's body defining beauty starting with the right side of the brain were the word is located. The position of B, E, A, U, T, I, F, U, L, etc.,
6. The numerical number is reflected on interfaces devices etc. The binary value is automatically calculated as well and displayed.
7. Lastly the light wave or acoustic is compiled and played on devices etc.

So, a single word will have seven meanings all in different locations.

Ideally is for all to send the results of the thinking back to a central command.

In the Brain language word-sequencing construction of the word beauty. This involves other factors you must consider. Beauty is in the eyes of the beholder. This is true here.

1. Right back side.
2. Right eye.
3. Left eye.
4. Beauty describes the face that starts where the hair begins and ends etc. in line with the chin.
    So, this becomes part of the language.
5. The cheeks define beauty as part of the smile. So smiling is part of the sequence.
6. A quick smile.
7. A left-eye wink.

Brain-specific language construction rules.

1. Every word must start with a specific reference point in the brain where the word is stored. e.g. right back side. It should be noted that some words are stored on the right backside of the brain while others like woman, her, herself, etc. are stored on the left back side. Some, like the president, are stored centrally on top of the brain.

2. Each word must have 7 basic expressions: written language, [EEG, MEGG, fMRI scans,] alphabetical body map, numerical and binary body map, sound waves as spoken words, electromagnetic or light waves, and brain language sequencing.

3. Each word in the brain language sequence must have an end which is a deflation situation where things go to normal. That means every beginning except in other situations must start with an opening; usually a position in the brain where the word is stored and must end with deflate or shoulders down or calm down. More like a full stop.

4. Alphabetical order must be on the body down to the legs.

5. The numerical order number in the map must be on the back of the body down to the legs.

6. Every or most body sequence expression of a word must include the place in the brain where the word is stored; the vibrations and in which of the two ears. Must include the motor neuron commands sent to the body by the brain. Must include the body parts in reference. Must include actions and the resultant effect and what happens to the resultant effect after. Must have an end e.g. deflate or calm down.

7. Some words can be constructed without a reference point but with a direct reference to the organs. The brain does not store the words like legs in the brain but directly in the legs themselves.

8. The brain stores words either on the right side of the brain or the left side. But every word is a mirror-image word in one of the 7 expressions. That means if a word like think is on the right side of the brain there is a mirror image of the same word but in a different form on the left side of the brain.

9. Whether speaking or thinking the tongue is involved as it creates words as sound waves that are bounced to the correct position in the brain where the word is stored but reflected straight away to the opposite side of the brain where a different format is stored and bounced back to the tongue. This means in constructing the words like thinking this might involve the actual bouncing of the words on the tongue, then to the position the word is stored, then to the opposite side of the brain, and back again to the tongue.

10. Some words involve rotational properties. The construction of words like rotate must include the actual rotation. This is enabled by the rotary propeller. I will explain this in detail in the next book.

11. Some words will be command words like sit, stop, stand, etc. and all these must have two meanings. Sitting as a written word. Sitting as a definition of the body using alphabetical order. The actual sitting, where one must sit down. This is easily achieved by recording a person sitting down and using acoustic or electromagnetic waves to create the meaning where one says sit. The body movements involved in sitting happen. See the example of this definition of the command to raise one's hand where the person raises his hand but without knowing it.

https://www.youtube.com/watch?v=MeJzkiv577Q

12. Some word definitions involve facial movements, for example, smile. This is possible as at the beginning we can

record a person smiling, the actual facial movements. Then store this so that when one says smile, we can have this as part of the definition of smile. The actual physical process; the movement of the face.

13. The language must distinguish between gender by separating where words like man, he, himself are stored i.e. in the right back side and words referring to feminine are stored on the left back side.

I will elaborate on this in the next book.

So far, we have covered.

1. Brain language construction.
2. Brain region classification.
3. Brain word mapping. I can only add that in the end we will create a map of all the words as places where they are stored by the brain. It is possible to write which sections of the brain is used to store all words even above 20 000 words.
4. Brain word sequencing.
5. Language dictionary. We must be able to come up with a dictionary of each word and all its 7 expressions. That means each word will have 7 meanings all in one place. If one is to check what clap means; he or she will be shown the written word, the spelling, and where in the body the letters are stored. The number equivalent and the binary equivalent. The spectrogram. The sound waves. The electromagnetic and acoustic waves. The EEG, MEG, PET, and fMRI scans and the brain language sequencing.
6. Body language alphabet.
7. Numbers body mapping.
8. Language construction rules.

9. The recording and processing of the sound and light waves.
10. Mirror image and reverse mirror image.
11. Oscillations in the third person.

The Comprehensive Approach.

Comprehensive Approach

Benchmark +   Other Methods = Ideal Methods

Benchmark	Other Methods
Brain Language	Electroencephalogram
Acoustic Wave	
Sound Wave	Magnetoencephalography
Brain Word Atlas	Functional Magnetic Resonance Imaging (fMRI)
Body Alphabet Map	
Body Color & Number Mapping	Positron Emission Tomography (PET)
Converting words to numbers then to binary	
Binary to device commands	

As I said, treat this method as the benchmark for decoding the brain. One which you can evaluate your project if you are doing the right thing. This should not work as a substitute for your project. I know the effort and sweat put in and endured. So, use this method as a litmus test to test what you are doing. This method works and I believe it will be the only future method of decoding the brain. The ideal comprehensive method will include this method and all modern and scientific methods you are currently using. I have created a lot of brain language templates that really work so use these to test your results. I urge you to compare what you have and what I have uploaded on SoundCloud.

https://soundcloud.com/david-gomadza

If you need anything let me know I can upload anything, commands that work, other words,

 etc.

info@twofuture.world

davidomadza@otmail.com

https://twitter.com/DGomadza

https://www.youtube.com/@davidgomadza6875

So, at the end of the day the ideal method is this benchmark plus whatever you are doing. This is the future.

I think what you should all do is use these templates and samples which are already accurate and defined then use these to test your subjects knowing that what you have is tested hence what you get will be definite and accurate results.

Body Zoning.

The whole body must be zoned into diamond shapes that are later color coded using the following colors: gold, blue, purple, and scarlet. When that is done the zone number, the color, and the function of that area of the body, the organs, and the sensory activities are all linked to areas of the brain responsible for these. Also, the commands and actions involved are all linked as a template.

Let us take the heart for example.

Just as an example in the diagram below the heart is marked by the color purple and can be classified as four across and two down.

This is noted and it is linked to the part of the brain linked to its control and all other areas involved like the blood vessels. This must also be linked to the points on the spinal cord where the motor codes exit and enter.

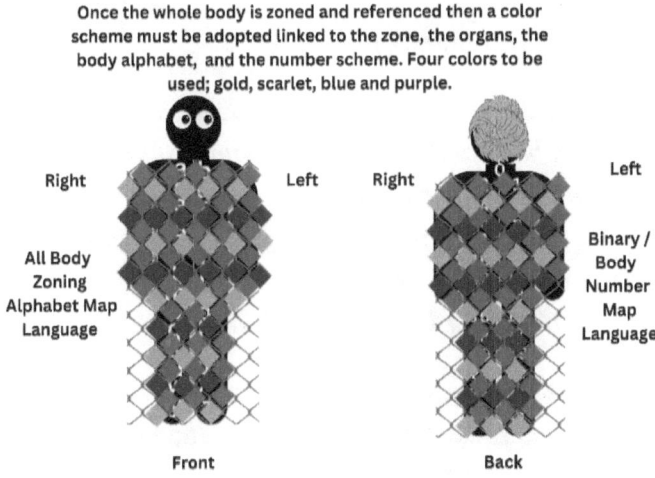

Once the whole body is zoned and referenced then a color scheme must be adopted linked to the zone, the organs, the body alphabet, and the number scheme. Four colors to be used; gold, scarlet, blue and purple.

A digital color-coded chest armor.

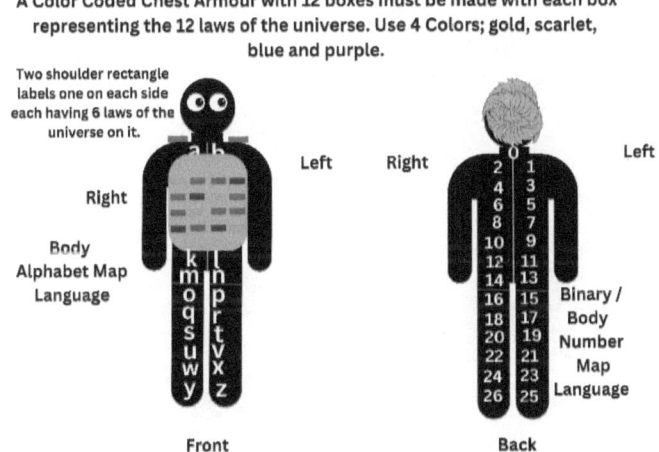

A Color Coded Chest Armour with 12 boxes must be made with each box representing the 12 laws of the universe. Use 4 Colors; gold, scarlet, blue and purple.

As part of zoning the body, a digital chest armor must be created with 12 boxes. Each box must have one of the 12 laws of the universe linked to the function of the part of that body.

This is also linked to the 7 senses of the body.

Sensory integration is the neurological process that organizes sensations from one's body and from the environment and makes it possible to use the body to make adaptive responses within the environment. To do this, the brain must register, select, interpret, compare, and associate sensory information in a flexible, constantly changing pattern. (A Jean Ayres, 1989).

Sensory Integration is the adequate and processing of sensory stimuli in the central nervous system – the brain. It enables us to interact with our environment appropriately.

Wikipedia.

Sensory processing is the brain's process of receiving, interpreting, and organizing input from all the active senses at any given moment. If the processing in the central nervous system is incorrect, an appropriate, goal-oriented, and planned reaction is not possible.

7 Senses.

Sight

Visual perception is the process of comparing visual stimuli to past experiences. Visual perception is divided into five areas: motor coordination, figure-ground perception, form constancy, position in space, and spatial relations.

Smell is interpreted by the brain through vibrations.

Taste is the ability to detect the taste of substances.

Hearing

Hearing is the ability to perceive sound by detecting vibrations, changes in pressure, and differentiating sound stimuli. The auditory system differentiates between localization, differentiation, and log/lock.

Touch is a perception caused by the activation of neural receptors in the skin, hair follicles, and pressure receptors.

Vestibular

The vestibular system helps us coordinate our eye movements, balance, equilibrium, and language.

Proprioception

Proprioception is the sense of relative position and strength of effort in movement, allowing us to plan our movements without vision.

Aerial View of the head

**An EEG 10-10 International system
can be superimposed on top and all
linked to the zones created below**

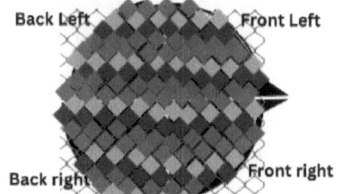

Back Left   Front Left

Back right   Front right

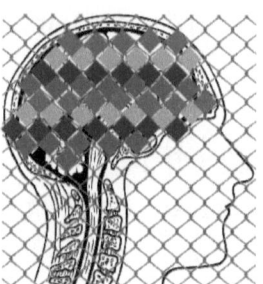

**The whole head is number-marked, zoned
and color coded using 4 colors; gold, blue, purple
and scarlet and equal diamond shapes**

Converting Words Into Numbers & Binary

Clap = c.l.a.p = 3.12.1.16 = 1100010010000100010110

Start = s.t.a.r.t = 19.20.1.18.20 = 110010010000000010001100000100000

Stop = s.t.o.p = 19.20.15.16 = 110010010000000001010100010110

David = d.a.v.i.d = 4.1.22.9.4 = 10000010010001010010100

Brain = b.r.a.i.n = 2.18.1.9.14 = 10000110000001100100010100

Characters and their binary value.

Lower Case.

Brain Code. The Benchmark of Decoding the Brain.

a: 01100001

b: 01100010

c: 01100011

d: 01100100

e: 01100101

f: 01100110

g: 01100111

h: 01101000

i: 01101001

j: 01101010

k: 01101011

l: 01101100

m: 01101101

n: 01101110

o: 01101111

p: 01110000

q: 01110001

r: 01110010

s: 01110011

t: 01110100

u: 01110101

v: 01110110

w: 01110111

x: 01111000

y: 01111001

z: 01111010

Uppercase.

A: 01000001

B: 01000010

C: 01000011

D: 01000100

E: 01000101

F: 01000110

G: 01000111

H: 01001000

I: 01001001

J: 01001010

K: 01001011

L: 01001100

M: 01001101

Brain Code. The Benchmark of Decoding the Brain.

N: 01001110

O: 01001111

P: 01010000

Q: 01010001

R: 01010010

S: 01010010

T: 01010010

U: 01010101

V: 01010110

W: 01010111

X: 01011000

Y: 01011001

Z: 01011010N: 01001110

Start 192011820

Stop 19201516

Clap 312116

Sit 19920

Stand 19201144

Jump 10211316

Rotate

Lift

Drop

Sing

Shout

Cough

See

Read

Write

Sleep

Open

Close

Hit

Dumb

Initialize

End

Restart

Quick

Slow

Swallow

Fast

Run

Squat

Sneeze

Cough

Inhale

Exhale

Turn

Point

Finger

Leg

Arm

Hand

Shoulder

Stomach

Heart

Liver

Converting more words into numbers then into binary.

1. Collar 3151212118
2. Analyze 11411225265
3. Fan 6114
4. Whack 2381311
5. Shoot 198151520
6. Maul 1312112
7. Generate 75145181205
8. Led 1254
9. Expose 5241615195
10. Scruff 193182166
11. Repulse 185162112195
12. File
13. Define
14. Sculpt
15. Prove
16. Gather
17. Direct
18. Scrawl
19. Initiate
20. Reorganize
21. Prepare
22. Imitate
23. Cure
24. Manage
25. Maim
26. Structure
27. Hitch
28. Spur
29. Meet
30. Bow
31. Collide
32. Hurtle
33. Advocate
34. Mock
35. Remove

36. Pummel
37. Derive
38. Systematize
39. Obtain
40. Listen   1291920514
41. Appropriate
42. Abscond
43. Bathe
44. Log
45. Link
46. Advance
47. Campaign
48. Mimic
49. Rock
50. Hang
51. Lurch
52. Sprint
53. Rebuild
54. Pirate
55. Lose
56. Kick
57. Slug
58. Bushwhack
59. Patrol
60. Turn off
61. Dash
62. Emerge
63. Distinguish
64. Restore
65. Stimulate
66. Divert
67. Slay
68. Resign
69. Vacate
70. Save
71. Flog
72. Spike

73. Tape
74. Master
75. Assemble
76. Hasten
77. Install
78. Learn
79. Itemize
80. Collaborate
81. Brighten
82. Convert
83. Gain
84. Edge
85. Observe
86. Rob
87. Tug
88. Eat
89. Contract
90. Submit
91. Synthesize
92. Snitch
93. Check
94. Order
95. Sustain
96. Sense
97. Educate
98. Step
99. Race
100. Effectually

Mouth

Teeth

Tongue

Lips

Saliva

Glands

Stomach

Intestine

Gallbladder

Kidney

Ureter

Bladder

Ureter

Ovaries

Uterus

Cervix

Placenta

Vulva

Vagina

Testicles

Prostrate

Penis

Scrotum

Creating the acoustic wave alphabetical order.

The question that kept coming to mind was this; Can we create an alphabetic order of thoughts? Can we create an acoustic wave alphabetical order from A to Z when a person is only thinking about letters of the alphabet?
Great news. The answer is yes.
Hear it first-hand. Worlds first.

https://soundcloud.com/david-gomadza

Yes, we can write the alphabetical order of sounds the brain language understands as A to Z.
This is the breakthrough.
This means just like the English language we can construct the language of the brain from the alphabetical order.
The way we have mapped the alphabetical order on the body will come handy here. The system identifies the letters in alphabetical order. But the question is that since we can simply create a word from the letters of the alphabetic order does the bringing together of C, L, A, and P form the word Clap as understood by the brain?
Can we join the electromagnetic or acoustic wave letters to build an acoustic or electromagnetic wave word that the brain will recognize as a word?
The first answer is yes to some extent. But after modifying this word according to the brain language rules, we have introduced then it becomes a **big yes**.

Just like DNA our brains when creating word classification and language sequences; use similar principles. That means each body sequence or word definition must have a start.
Remember what the start is?

The position in the brain where the brain stores the word. On The right back side, we can call this from now on RBS.

In addition, language sequences must have an end. In most cases Deflation. Which I can define as a return to the initial position or a calm position where shoulders are dropped down.

I have created these two parts of the body language sequencing. So now we can start our word construction. Explain why this is important?

If a person thinks about clapping or if someone speaks the word clap. The brain first will locate the position it has stored the word in the brain. Right back side. Now we can construct the word. C, L, A, P then add the deflate.

Now the brain if the person thinks about the word clap now will locate the place it stores the word. Then the place on the body where c is, then l, then a, and lastly p. Then it deflates as an end more like a full stop in sentence writing.

Now we compare the sound waves [MP3] and the light or electromagnetic waves together with the spectrograms to see if the waves when the person speaks the word clap, and when he thinks about the word and the word we have constructed are the same first; or understood as a command by the brain.

https://soundcloud.com/david-gomadza

This is the clap I have created.

Recall the brain stored words in either one of the four regions of the brain. This word clap is stored on the right back side.

Every word therefore in the brain language has a start and an end that is like a full stop in English language.

So, CLAP is constructed this way.

CLAP = Right back side + C + L + A + P + deflate.

This is the result.

https://www.youtube.com/watch?v=hdwaiJ7JiGE

The system recognizes the word as an acoustic wave even though noise has affected this and the fact that a recording has silent places that need trimming as well.

I can say outright that this works.

That means we do not even need to test and record words from the brain.

Now we can simply refine our alphabetical order and use our brain language construction to create any word on earth as a brain language.

Ladies and gentlemen this is the breakthrough you have been **waiting for.**

Congratulations humanity, you can now start talking with thoughts. This is now possible from now and forever.

We can simply construct the language of the brain.

Thank you. I am your Global President for a reason.

Constructing Brain Commands.

We can use the same idea to construct commands the brain understands. Instead of telling the brain to spell the word. We can ask the brain to perform the commands.

We can construct all commands that tell the body to perform such an activity. We can create motor neuron commands that work.

We know how the brain works. Our language construction can help us create commands to lift hands, to turn around to sit, to stand, to open the mouth, to sleep, to imagine having sex, to have arousal, to feel hungry, to bend down, to run, to curse with the middle finger. I mean everything. This means we can create sound waves that tell the brain to lift the arm with the body lifting the arm.

Believe me, we have reached that stage.

We can make these commands that can be used with anyone with injuries etc.

Visit SoundCloud to search for all tracks that have lift arm, leg, or all these are **motor neuron commands**.

https://soundcloud.com/david-gomadza

Watch this video.
If this does not work for you it means not amplified enough for you. So, ask your subjects. This works. I have tested it.

https://www.youtube.com/watch?v=MeJzkiv577Q

Imagine how many people need to move their arms but they cannot due to injuries, disability, etc. Now from today, we can do all that. But some people will need some devices that make this happen. But feel free to try this to work for you. Or test on people you know are unable to do this.

The greatest breakthrough of the century if you ask me.

We can ask the brain to think about feelings, moods, and all kinds of experiences. All that is needed is playing an mp3 to take someone from sadness to happiness. Imagine a world where we make people feel good. This is no longer a mystic thing in the religious circle, no. We can make anyone experience any kind of mood.
Watch these videos. Make sure your arms are beside your body and not holding anything. Make sure you have enough room.

https://www.youtube.com/watch?v=4ontY0ed6GE

https://www.youtube.com/watch?v=KeTMUMgDw6c

Check this out but only for those above 18.

https://www.youtube.com/watch?v=ay1f5zP5oZE

I will expand on this subject in volume VI.

To be continued…

APPLICATION FOR A PATENT FOR A ROBOT THAT IS AS GOOD AS A HUMAN BEING AND THE OPERATING SYSTEM IS SOFTWARE BASED ON THIS INVENTION.

The brain language and everything contained in all books, the soundwaves, acoustic waves, and electromagnetic waves on Soundcloud, YouTube [LINKS BELOW] and everything to be created **by** me.

Namely:

Decoding the Brain. The Manual and Guiding Principles.
David Gomadza.
ISBN 978-1-4477-6542-4

Volume VI.

Brain Code.
The Benchmark of Decoding the Brain. One Against which all are Evaluated.

David Gomadza

ISBN 978-1-4477-6925-5

Volume V.

Genesis. Brain Language Construction in Progress. Breakthrough in Decoding the Brain.

David Gomadza
ISBN 978-1-4477-8931-4

Volume IV.

DATESTAMP:28 March 2022 Thoughts to Word or Audio.

David Gomadza

ISBN 978-1-4477-9760-9

Volume III

Decoding Thoughts and Inner Voice.: Explanations and Debunking

the Misconceptions.

David Gomadza
ISBN 979-8801455488

Volume II

Thoughts to Word or Audio: How to Know Exactly What

Someone Is Thinking.

David Gomadza
ISBN 979-8703923498

Volume I

This patent is an addition to the patents in all the mentioned above books.

This patent is specific to a human-like robot.

The robot will use the brain decoding invention in this book. The operating system will use the invention in this book in such a way that it will be as clever as a human being and will perform tasks, movements, etc. as good as a human being. Will talk and process information faster than any other currently existing robots.
The commands for these robots will be constructed using the alphabetic order, body language sequencing, and all methods in the

above books. The invention in this book uses all invented expressions and forms of a single word. The robot will be so intelligent because it will use the following 7 expressions of any word to process information fast.

1. The English or any other language's written form.
2. Brain language sequencing which was invented in this book.
3. The body alphabetical order map I invented in all the books.
4. The numerical body maps.
5. The sound wave that is spoken word.
6. The electromagnetic waves and the acoustic waves.
7. Lastly the spectrogram and all EEG, MEG, PET, and fMRI scans.

This is what will make it faster as it can easily understand any word in seven different forms making it intelligent. This will be part of its operating software which we will develop.

We will use the acoustic alphabetical order created to generate commands like asking the robot to sit, raise its hand, raise its head, jump etc.

Some of the commands can be viewed on YouTube and the alphabetic order in acoustic or electromagnetic waves is on Soundcloud.

Follow these links.

https://soundcloud.com/david-gomadza

https://www.youtube.com/watch?v=KeTMUMgDw6c

https://www.youtube.com/watch?v=4ontY0ed6GE

https://www.youtube.com/watch?v=MeJzkiv577Q

The design of the robot will use human proportions.
The details of which can be expanded on request if need be.

Signed
David Gomadza
Date 03/04/2023
davidomadza@otmail.com

Get the next volume.

Decoding the Brain. The Manual and Guiding Principles.
David Gomadza.
ISBN 978-1-4477-6542-4

Volume VI.

Signed
David Gomadza
03/04/2023
First Global President of The World
info@twofuture.world
www.twofuture.world